Under the Wings of Rafa'el

BLESSINGS, SONGS, AND
EXPLORATIONS
FOR A HEALING PATH

~

Sharon Bernstein

Editor: Andrew Ramer

Designer: Ellen Toomey

Cover Art: "Raffaele" by Carlo Bertè, 2000, www.carloberte.it

Companion recordings available for download or on CD.
Please visit www.sharonbernstein.com/under-the-wings-of-rafael

Table of Contents

Author's Note

Under the Wings of Rafa'el began as an impromptu set of prayers with recordings and supplementary materials for a congregant who had been diagnosed with cancer. My desire was to create a journey, for the congregant as well as her partner, that would support her during her treatment, provide tools for spiritual connection and growth, and help make the time one of anticipation, enrichment, and even a little fun. For each of her twelve medical treatments, I chose a prayer (some specifically associated with healing, others concentrating on the body and spirit), recorded it, wrote some thoughts, meditations, and exercises designed to enhance the congregant's experience of the prayer, and then sent it all as a packet the night before the treatment.

What you see here is quite different from the original set of materials. Some of the prayers and music are different and the exploratory thoughts are expanded far beyond the original tiny booklet that I had conceived. Creating this journey became a journey in and of itself: a bringing together and traversing of many paths on which I have walked, and the many glorious people, teachers, learnings, and practices I've encountered upon them. There is a bit of each of them in here: their gifts of healing and mindfulness, prayer, Judaism, art, music, and science. Above all, this project bears the imprint of the people with whom I have had the privilege of sharing life's sacred moments. It is to you that this book is dedicated.

INTRODUCTION

According to Jewish tradition, there are four angels who watch over us as we go to sleep at night. Sometimes I imagine them: Micha'el on our right, bathing us in holiness; Gavri'el on our left, infusing us with strength; Uri'el in front, sprinkling light on the road ahead; and Rafa'el at our back, immensely soft, protective wings holding and sheltering us, particularly in times of healing.

What those times of healing are, and what the idea of healing itself is, can vary greatly. Healing can sometimes mean looking towards and achieving a cure. It can also mean finding some measure of comfort, peace, contentment or wholeness when a cure is not clear or possible. Within the context of this book, I see healing as an exploration, an experiencing, of our circumstances and ourselves within them, and of finding and creating paths that provide us with sustenance and support.

In the pages that follow you will find an experiential healing journey, structured as a series of twelve prayers with supporting materials in the form of music and meditations, explorations, and artistic exercises. These prayers were chosen and the supporting materials were designed to help those of us in a time of healing to reflect on what we are experiencing, providing new options for looking at ourselves and the world around us through a kaleidoscope of possibilities.

The prayers included here are in Hebrew, and were selected from a rich body of sacred texts handed down by the Jewish tradition. But it is not necessary to be of a particular faith or religious practice to journey with them, as these texts and ideas can all be approached as metaphors, adapting to our individual understandings of and relationships with the universe.

In this, and in all your journeys, I wish you r'fuah sh'leimah: full healing, however we each define healing in this moment, of the body, mind, and spirit, speedily and soon.

GUIDE

What Is In Here?

There are twelve sections in this journey, each corresponding to a different theme and prayer. Within each section are the following three elements:

TEXT
the text in its original Hebrew with English transliteration and translation

EXPLORATIONS
meditations, ponderings, imagery, and exercises inspired by the text of the prayer

RECORDING
a musical setting of the text, available separately on CD or digital download

There is also a short appendix at the end of the book, which you can refer to at any time. It includes information on the power of imagery, the texts and how to pronounce them, the structure of Hebrew blessings, what I call "God-language" (how we refer to God), and some background on the music.

How to Use These Materials

The twelve sections and the materials within them are modular: designed to be used in a variety of ways, and in any order you like.

You may want to do a section a day, a section a week, or turn to the book when you feel called to it. Some people have chosen an individual prayer to go along with each stage of a medical treatment. To get started you can:

- Start at the beginning, with the first prayer.

- Open the book at random and see where you find yourself.

- Read through the list of prayers found in the Table of Contents and go to one whose title calls out to you.

If something works for you, go with it. If not, skip it and move to another section. This is your journey — make it yours.

$$\sim$$

When you have selected a prayer, you can try some of the following possibilities, as you are able:

- Read the text and notice how it feels: physically, mentally, and spiritually.

- Explore the Explorations: in the order presented, or in any order you like.

- Listen to the recording — once or set to play repeatedly in a loop.

- Listen to the recording while reading the text.

  – Does the music impact your experience of the text?

  – Does the text impact your experience of the music?

- Sing or hum along with the recording
  (*If singing isn't an option, you can touch the music player*)

  – Sense the vibrations rippling through your body.

  – Do you feel vibrations more in one part of your body than another?

  – Try sending the vibrations to a particular part of your body, and see what it feels like.

- Make up your own chant for the text, letting words and sounds emerge from your throat spontaneously as you feel them.

- Write your own text or prayer along the theme of one of the prayers here or along a different theme of your choosing.

When you have experienced one prayer, you can move on to another one, as you feel called to do so. You may find that going through the whole series works for you, and you may also find that one prayer and the explorations that go along with it become a particular companion on your journey.

Again, there is no one right way to use this book and these prayers. They are yours.

∼

About the Explorations

The explorations are a beginning point: different ways of experiencing the words and ideas of each prayer that can lead in all kinds of directions (including new explorations). While the explorations are each included in a particular section, you may find that they work in other sections as well, either in their current forms, or slightly adjusted in content. Those that involve movement or additional materials are enclosed in a box, and can be done literally or in the mind's eye (or both). The explorations that are more in the form of questions and imagery can inspire mental meanderings, or writing, or both.

For Groups

If you're using *Under the Wings of Rafael* in a group, you can choose to all explore the same prayer at the same time, or have each person in the group focusing on whichever prayers they like. Group interactions could include, for example:

- Sharing thoughts, writings, or materials that emerge from the explorations.

- Using explorations as guided meditations, with a group leader or member reading the exploration aloud.

- Doing one of the drawing exercises as a group, either with everyone working together on one large piece of paper, or on a single sheet passed around, with each person adding something.

- Together creating new explorations, exercises, music, or texts on one or more of the themes.

SHEHECHEYANU (LIFE)

Text: Talmud Pesachim 7b, Sukkah 46a, and B'rachot 37b, 44a, and 59a
Melody: Sharon Bernstein

Baruch Atah Adonai,

Eloheinu Melech Ha-olam

She-he-che-yanu v'-ki-y'-manu

v'-hi-gi-yanu laz-man ha-zeh.

בָּרוּךְ אַתָּה יְיָ,

אֱלֹהֵינוּ מֶלֶךְ הָעוֹלָם,

שֶׁהֶחֱיָנוּ וְקִיְּמָנוּ

וְהִגִּיעָנוּ לַזְּמַן הַזֶּה.

Bountiful are You,

Who pours life into us,

supports and nurtures us,

and gathers us up into this moment.

Explorations

Take a moment . . .

and notice this moment,
whatever moment this moment may be.

Notice what's happening inside you, and outside you
Bring your attention from one point to another, within and with-out,
Gently feeling each point, allowing it to sink in,

Radiating through you, through your being,
Utterly and completely gathered up into

This moment.

~

1

Shehecheyanu is a prayer of beginnings, recited on the occasion of something new: the beginning of a holiday, the first time on a particular adventure, the achieving of an accomplishment, the first nectarine of the season. . .

Are there things that you are beginning at this time? Is there anything that is new? Is there something that you are revisiting but feels new,
or that you would like to feel new?

∾

What do the words "support" and "nurture" invoke for you? What would feel supporting at this time? What would feel nurturing?

As you enter into this journey, notice what supports and nurtures you — what gives you energy, relief, joy, and rest — inside you and in the world around you.

∾

Take a piece of paper and some colored pencils, pens, or paints.

Bring to mind something, internal or external, that nurtures and/or supports you.

Holding the image of that something in your mind, pick a color, and, either half-closing your eyes or closing them completely, make a free form drawing.

The drawing does not need to be representative — it can be more a drawing of the nurturing/supporting feeling.

Mostly, try letting the color go where it wants, enjoying the movement, the feeling of the pen (or pencil or paintbrush or crayon) on the paper.

∾

Now, bring to mind something else that supports/nurtures you.

If it was something external the last time, it could be internal this time. Or not. Your choice.

Pick a color. It can be the same color or a different color.

Holding the image of this something else in your mind, again do a free form drawing, on top of the other one.

Pay attention only to the feeling of the drawing, not how it's interacting with the first drawing. When you're done, you can look, see how it feels.

If you like, keep going with additional drawing, either on the same page or on different pages.

∾

This prayer ends with the words: *v'higiyanu lazman hazeh* — who gathers us up into this moment. When possible, notice the moment you're in, feeling its fullness, its richness, along with whatever loveliness or challenge that might be in it.

Min Hameitzar (Widening)

Text: Psalms 118:5
Melody: folk

Min ha-meitzar karati Yah,

Anani va-merchav Yah.

מִן הַמֵּצַר קָרָאתִי יָּה,

עָנָנִי בַמֶּרְחָב יָהּ.

Out of the narrow place of distress, I called to Yah,

Who responded by widening.

Explorations

Imagine, for a moment, calling out:
A sensation in your heart, your mind, your throat, your body.

How does it feel?

∾

In this prayer, there is a calling out, but no request for a response.

Do you feel a difference between calling out and asking for a response?

And do you feel a difference between asking for a response, and receiving a response?

Could asking for a response be a form of receiving a response?

∾

Is there anything that you would like to ask for now?
If yes, what kind of a response or responses would you like to receive?

～

What is the feeling of widening?

Is it a stretchy feeling?

Is it something that, once stretched, remains widened,
Like bubble gum or taffy?

Or is it something that reflexively returns to its previous state,
Like a rubber band?

Or is it perhaps like an accordion,
Something that you can widen and narrow at will?

～

Try some widening and narrowing movements,
In your mind's eye, or physically, as you are able.

First with your hands,
A little like playing the accordion.

Now the feeling expanding to your breath,
A sense of your sides widening out and coming back in.

Now the feeling expanding further,
Your entire body widening and narrowing.

Now, extend it beyond your physical self,
Feeling your essence, your spirit,
And all that is around you and in the world
Widening and narrowing.

While doing this, try to let go of any thoughts of arriving at a particular place. The
idea is more to play with possibility: exploring, expanding, and moving amongst
different modes of being and relating, with ourselves and the world around us.

ELOHAI N'SHAMAH (SOUL)

Text: Babylonian Talmud: B'rachot 60b, based on Kohelet 12:7
Melody: Rabbi Shefa Gold

Elo-hai,

N'-shamah she-natata bi

T'-horah hi.

אֱלֹהַי,

נְשָׁמָה שֶׁנָּתַתָּ בִּי

טְהוֹרָה הִיא.

Elohai,

The soul that you gifted me

Is pure.

Explorations

There is a mystical teaching that says that we have three parts to that which we call our soul:

nefesh: our body, our life force;

ruach: our wisdom, insight, awareness, and spirit;

n'shamah: a divine spark blown into us at birth.

～

Think for a moment about your soul.

Where do you imagine it residing?
Can you imagine it in different places in your body?

Try feeling it in your solar plexus,

in your heart,

in your left pinky,

in your ankles

in your whole body.

Wherever it is, imagine it sending forth light,
Illuminating every single part of you.

~

Inhale:

Breath flowing in . . .

. . . filling, nourishing, cleansing, revitalizing.

Exhale:

Breath flowing out . . .

. . . pouring, flowing, abundant releasing

~

Try sensing your soul as a gift.

Imagine it arriving, fabulously gift-wrapped, shiny paper and ribbons all over.

Open it, check out what's inside.

Explore all of its nooks and crannies as if you've never seen it before.
Never seen anything like it.

Like an amazing toy,
with buttons and levers and whirligigs,
moving parts and hidden compartments.
flowing silken rainbows, sweet chimes, and feathery softness,
twinkly lights, playgrounds, and abundant gardens to explore . . .

The best gift. Ever.

ASHER YATZAR (BODY)

Text: Babylonian Talmud: B'rachot 60b; Melody: Sharon Bernstein

Ba-ruch a-tah A-do-nai	בָּרוּךְ אַתָּה יְיָ
Elo-hey-nu melech ha-olam,	אֱלֹהֵינוּ מֶלֶךְ הָעוֹלָם,
Asher yatzar et ha-adam b'-choch-mah,	אֲשֶׁר יָצַר אֶת הָאָדָם בְּחָכְמָה,
U-vara vo n'-ka-vim n'-ka-vim,	וּבָרָא בוֹ נְקָבִים נְקָבִים,
Cha-lu-lim cha-lu-lim,	חֲלוּלִים חֲלוּלִים,
Ga-lu-i v'-yadu-a	גָּלוּי וְיָדוּעַ
Lif-ney chi-sei ch'-vo-decha	לִפְנֵי כִסֵּא כְבוֹדֶךָ
She-im yi-pa-tei-ach e-chad mei-hem,	שֶׁאִם יִפָּתֵחַ אֶחָד מֵהֶם,
O yisa-teim e-chad mei-hem,	אוֹ יִסָּתֵם אֶחָד מֵהֶם,
I ef-shar l'-hit-kayeim	אִי אֶפְשַׁר לְהִתְקַיֵּים
v'-la-a-mod l'-fa-necha:	וְלַעֲמוֹד לְפָנֶיךָ:
Ba-ruch A-tah A-do-nai,	בָּרוּךְ אַתָּה יְיָ,
Ro-fei chol basar,	רוֹפֵא כָל בָּשָׂר,
U-mafli la-a-sot.	וּמַפְלִיא לַעֲשׂוֹת:

Bountiful are You,

Who fashioned the human body in wisdom,

Creating in us places that open,

And hollows that are enclosed.

How well you know

That if one of the hollows were to open,

Or one of the openings to close,

It would be impossible to go on.

Bountiful are You,

Healer of all bodies,

Wondrous in actions.

Explorations

What do you think is wise, cool, fabulous, *wow* about how our bodies were created?
What do you like about your body?
Are there any parts of your body that would cherish some extra care?

Take a moment, and give some care to those parts of your body . . .

> . . . breathe into them,
> . . . caress them (physically or mentally),
> . . . play with them (imagine them on a see-saw, or rocking out at a concert),
> . . . dunk them in love.

❧

The phrase "who fashioned the human body in wisdom" can be understood in (at least) two ways:

~ there was wisdom in how the human body and form was created
~ wisdom was instilled into our bodies.

> Do you feel wisdom in your body? If yes, where?

> > Might you feel it in more than one place?
> > Do you sense it as being woven into your fibers,
> > Diffused throughout you?
> > Or perhaps more focused in one place or another?
> > Can you move it around?

❧

N'kavim are openings —
    places where the inside of us can come into contact with the outside world.

      They can let things in
      And let things out.

          Are there things you would like to let in?
          And are there things you would you like to let out?

∽

Chalulim are enclosed hollows,
enfolding and protecting our inner parts such as the heart, the abdomen, the brain.

Is there anything — physical, mental, emotional —
that you are wanting to keep enclosed, safe, protected?

Do you, yourself, sometimes wish to feel enclosed, safe, protected?

∽

Take out some art supplies, and make a drawing of yourself (representative or abstract) that includes your physical openings and hollows.

Then, either making another drawing, or using another color on the same drawing, draw your mental, emotional, and spiritual openings and hollows.

Are there any places that are open that you would like to see more closed?

Are there any places that are closed that you would like to see more open?

~

Close your eyes for a moment,

Visualize your openings and closings.

Imagine them gently moving, shifting

Dancing into any place or position that you would like them to be in.

ELOHAI N'TZOR (SPEECH)

Text: Mar son of Ravina (4th century)
Melody: Sharon Bernstein

Elo-hai,

אֱלֹהַי,

N'-tzor l'-shoni mei-ra.

נְצוֹר לְשׁוֹנִי מֵרָע,

U-s'fa-tai mi-dabeir mir-mah.

וּשְׂפָתַי מִדַּבֵּר מִרְמָה.

P'-tach libi b'-tora-techa.

פְּתַח לִבִּי בְּתוֹרָתֶךָ.

Aseih l'ma-an sh'me-cha,

עֲשֵׂה לְמַעַן שְׁמֶךָ,

Aseih l'ma-an y'mi-necha,

עֲשֵׂה לְמַעַן יְמִינֶךָ,

Aseih l'ma-an k'dusha-techa.

עֲשֵׂה לְמַעַן קְדֻשָּׁתֶךָ.

Asieh l'ma-an tora-techa.

עֲשֵׂה לְמַעַן תּוֹרָתֶךָ.

Elohai,

Protect my tongue from speaking harmfully,

And my lips from uttering hurtful words.

Open my heart with your wisdom.

For the sake of your name,

For the sake of your strength,

For the sake of your holiness,

For the sake of your teachings.

Explorations

The term *lashon hara*, literally meaning "harmful speech", is often understood as the unkind things we may say about others. However, *lashon hara* can also be seen as the things we may say to ourselves, the non-constructive, and sometimes hurtful thoughts and words we direct inwards.

Are there ways in which your speech or words, out loud or inside yourself, have been harmful or an impediment to you?

Do you have words that you use towards or about yourself that are not useful?

What are some of these words or phrases?

~

Try taking a hurtful word that you may think or say about yourself, and imagine placing it on your tongue.

Now, first making sure that there is no one directly in front of you, do a good long raspberry or motorboat*, and let it slip away.

If that feels good, try it again with the same word or another,
or perhaps even a phrase.

* raspberry: also known as a bronx cheer, it involves sticking your tongue out, and, blowing air through it, making a sound like an outboard motor. A motorboat is doing the same thing with your lips. You can also try something like drop kicking the word/ phrase or sending it into outer space with a rocket.

~

The 4th line says: "open my heart with wisdom."

Imagine your heart opening and closing.

What does that opening look like, feel like?
Is it a gate? A window? A valve?
A sea anemone? A flower?

What rushes in? What rushes out?

~

Are there certain ideas, phrases, or words which are helpful to you:
Which help your heart to open,
That help you feel comfortable, supported, safe?

Try taking some of those helpful words, ideas, and phrases,
and place them in your tongue, lips, and mind,

And see what happens.

~

Elohai N'tzor is a prayer designed to express one's hopes and prayers
from the heart.

What are your hopes/wishes/dreams/prayers?

Do they change?

~

Take a moment (or many moments) to express, in any form you like
(single words, bullet points, poetry, collage, drawing, paint throwing . . .)

Something that represents some of your deepest prayers, hopes, dreams, wishes.

R'faeini (Heal Me)

Text: Jeremiah 17:14
Melody: Sharon Bernstein

R'fa-eini Adonai v'ei-rafei

Hoshi-eini v'-iva-shei-a.

רְפָאֵנִי יְהוָה וְאֵרָפֵא

הוֹשִׁיעֵנִי וְאִוָּשֵׁעָה.

Heal me, and I will heal.

Keep me safe, and I will be safe.

Explorations

What does the word "heal" invoke for you? What thoughts, feelings, desires?

Are there different kinds of healing for you?
What do they look like, feel like?

~

What does the word "safe" invoke for you? What thoughts, feelings, desires?

Are there different kinds of safety for you?
What do they look like, feel like?

~

Imagine yourself for a moment on a tightrope,
Teetering a little, afraid of falling,
Then falling and landing safely in a net
Soft as gossamer silk
Cushioned, fluffy, like a cloud.

Now imagine, in each and every moment,
That net beneath you, ready and waiting to catch you if you fall.

Helping you to feel absolutely, completely, safe.

～

Cup your hands in front of you.
This is your net.
Feel how light and strong it is.

Now gradually bring your hands apart from each other,
stretching and expanding the net,
weaving its tensile strength around and under you.

How does it feel?

～

Picture a cushy life preserver within easy reach,
In whatever shape or design you like:
Maybe covered with flowers, or pinstripes, or cartoons, or soft, sparkly yarn.

It's there for any time you want something to hold on to, to help keep you going.

～

There is a rhythm to this prayer,
a rocking, a back-and-forth: of being, receiving, and giving.

Feel yourself for a moment in this rocking:
Receiving healing energy from an external source
Then melding it with the healing energy from your internal source
The two joined energies intermingling and spilling back and forth,
Rocking, flowing, in harmony.

~

If you are able, make a gentle rocking motion with your body,
side to side, front to back, or circular.

You can use very small movements, almost imagined, or larger.

You can move your whole body,
or a part of your body at a time: your hands, hips, ankles, elbows, tummy. . .

See how this rocking feels: in the different parts, in different ways.

Then rest, and see if the movement continues a bit inside of you,

A buoyant healing energy rippling and gliding through you.

ELOHEI OZ (SOURCE OF STRENGTH)

Text: Siman Elyakim
Melody: traditional from Calcutta

Elo-hei oz t'-hi-lati	אֱלֹהֵי עֹז תְּהִלָּתִי
R'-fa-eini v'ei-rafei	רְפָאֵנִי וְאֵרָפֵא
V'-tein mar-pei l'-ma-cha-lati	וְתֶן מַרְפֵּא לְמַחֲלָתִי
L'-val a-mut v'-e-safeh	לְבַל אָמוּת וְאֶסָּפֶה
L'-cha odeh b'-odi chai	לְךָ אוֹדֶה בְּעוֹדִי חַי
B'-toch rei-ai v'-gam a-chai	בְּתוֹךְ רֵעַי וְגַם אַחַי
V'-arbeh ma-halal si-chi	וְאַרְבֶּה מַהֲלַל שִׂיחִי
B'-kol areiv v'-niv ya-feh	בְּקוֹל עָרֵב וְנִיב יָפֶה
Y'-shu-at-cha t'-vo-eini	יְשׁוּעָתְךָ תְּבוֹאֵנִי
V'-al rag-lai t'-ki-meini	וְעַל רַגְלַי תְּקִימֵנִי
B'-shu-vi od e-ley cha-ni	בְּשׁוּבִי עוֹד אֵלֶי כַנִּי
L'-to-vat-cha ani tso-feh	לְטוֹבָתְךָ אֲנִי צוֹפֶה
K'-shov ki rav k'-eiv libi	קְשׁוֹב כִּי רַב כְּאֵב לִבִּי
K'-eish bo-eir b'-toch kir-bi	כְּאֵשׁ בּוֹעֵר בְּתוֹךְ קִרְבִּי
V'-lo not-rah n'-sha-mah bi	וְלֹא נוֹתְרָה נְשָׁמָה בִּי
V'-cho-chi hu m'-od ra-feh	וְכֹחִי הוּא מְאֹד רָפֶה
Y'-hi na chas-d'-cha alai	יְהִי נָא חַסְדְּךָ עָלַי
L'-som-chei-ni b'-ma-ga-lai	לְסָמְכֵנִי בְּמַעְגָּלַי
V'-chol ya-mai v'-gam lei-lai	וְכָל יָמַי וְגַם לֵילַי
Aha-lel-cha b'-no-am peh.	אֲהַלֶּלְךָ בְּנֹעַם פֶּה

El, the strength and source of my praise, heal me and I will be healed.
Brush balm on my illness, that I not fade.

I will thank you as long as I live, amidst friends and community,
Abundant praise will flower in my speech, with sweet voice and comely phrase.

May you bring me to safety and set me strong upon my limbs,
With your treasured help, I foresee returning to my place.

Please listen, for my heart hurts terribly, like a fire burning within me,
My spirits are low, my energy depleted.

May your lovingkindness be with me, supporting me on my journey,
And all my days as well as my nights,
My lips will be filled with praise to you.

Explorations

Are you experiencing any pain?

What kind of pain is it? Is it physical? Emotional? Both?

What is your relationship with the pain?
Do you accept it? Fear it? Fight it? Interact with it? All of the above?
Are there times that the pain is greater, or lesser?
Or more present, or more distant?

~

Take a moment to give some space and attention to your pain.
Then gently shift your attention elsewhere,
Then turn your attention again to your pain,
Then allow your attention to move elsewhere,
And continue shifting your noticing, back and forth.

As you do this,
See how it feels to interact with your pain in this way,
Whether it expands your sense of possibilities.

~

Imagine your legs as trees:
Thick, strong, vibrant;
Roots delving into and absorbing the richness of the earth.

Now imagine your tree-ness flowing upward,
Through your middle,
Extending out through your shoulders, elbows, wrists,
Leaves growing upon your fingers,
Stretching and unfurling to gather in sun and air.

Now up through your neck and crown,
Face upturned to the sky.
Life force rippling from roots to crown,
Toes through head, then down, then back up again.

Nourishment of sun, air, and earth
Refreshing, feeding, supporting
You.

~

Let's try a praise exercise.

Take a sheet of paper and pen you like, any color.

Now think of someone or something you like or admire. It can be anything: a person, object, part of nature, animal, book, movie, food – anything at all.

Now write, as a stream of consciousness, all of the praise you can come up with, focusing on the someone or something you have chosen.

When you have finished, look through what you have written, and allow the praise to fill you, glowingly burnishing every part of your mind and body.

El Na R'fa Na Lah (Heal Us)

Text: adapted from Bamidbar (Numbers) 12:13
Melody: folk

Eil na r'-fa na lah,

Eil na r'-fa na lo,

Eil na r'-fa na li,

Eil na r'-fa na lanu.

אֵל נָא רְפָא נָא לָהּ,

אֵל נָא רְפָא נָא לוֹ,

אֵל נָא רְפָא נָא לִי,

אֵל נָא רְפָא נָא לָנוּ.

El, please, heal her, please,

El, please, heal him, please,

El, please, heal me, please,

El, please, heal us, please.

Explorations

The first line of this prayer is the earliest Jewish prayer, recited by Moses on behalf of his sister, Miriam.

> There can be something powerful, potent,
> in reciting healing prayers for others,
> As well as having others recite prayers for us.

Take a moment now to send some prayers of healing to others.

And in that same moment, feel yourself receiving others' healing prayers as well.

~

As you chant or listen to the words of this prayer,
Allow a warm glow to enter your body:

Embracing,
Cradling,
Soothing

All of your insides,
Your organs, your cells, your blood, your mind,
Bringing life, healing, and rejuvenation,

Easing away anything unwanted or unnecessary.

~

Imagine a troupe of pacmen*, pacwomen, or pacpeople with wings, happily galavanting around inside you and gobbling up anything harmful or unuseful.

~

Draw – by hand or using a computer – a pac-angel with wings.

~

Vividly imagine your body strong, active, vibrant, responsive,
Adapting, as needed, to any changes.

* Pacman is an old video game in which a smiley-face gobbles up dots and monsters.
  As an alternative, you can use the image of any cheerfully munching creature, real
  or fiction.

Hashkiveinu (Safety)

Text: Babylonian Talmud B'rachot 4b
Melody: Sharon Bernstein

Hashki-veinu Adonai Elo-heynu l'-shalom,	הַשְׁכִּיבֵנוּ יְיָ אֱלֹהֵינוּ לְשָׁלוֹם,
V'-ha-ami-deinu mal-keinu l'-cha-yim.	וְהַעֲמִידֵנוּ מַלְכֵּנוּ לְחַיִּים.
U-f'-ros a-leinu sukat sh'-lo-mecha	וּפְרוֹשׁ עָלֵינוּ סֻכַּת שְׁלוֹמֶךְ
V'-tak-neinu b'-ei-tzah to-vah mi-l'-fa-necha,	וְתַקְּנֵנוּ בְּעֵצָה טוֹבָה מִלְּפָנֶיךָ,
V'-hoshi-einu l'-ma-an sh'-mecha.	וְהוֹשִׁיעֵנוּ לְמַעַן שְׁמֶךָ.
V'-ha-gein ba-a-deinu, v'-ha-seir mei-a-leinu	וְהָגֵן בַּעֲדֵנוּ, וְהָסֵר מֵעָלֵינוּ
O-yeiv, de-ver, v'-che-rev, v'-ra-av, v'-ya-gon,	אוֹיֵב, דֶּבֶר, וְחֶרֶב, וְרָעָב, וְיָגוֹן,
V'-ha-seir sa-tan mi-l'-fa-neynu u-mei-acha-reinu,	וְהָסֵר שָׂטָן מִלְּפָנֵינוּ וּמֵאַחֲרֵנוּ,
U-v'-tzeil k'-na-fecha tas-ti-reinu.	וּבְצֵל כְּנָפֶיךָ תַּסְתִּירֵנוּ.
Ki eil shom-reinu u-matzi-leinu a-tah,	כִּי אֵל שׁוֹמְרֵנוּ וּמַצִּילֵנוּ אָתָּה,
Ki eil me-lech cha-nun v'-ra-chum a-tah,	כִּי אֵל מֶלֶךְ חַנּוּן וְרַחוּם אָתָּה,
U-sh'-mor tzei-teinu u-vo-einu,	וּשְׁמוֹר צֵאתֵנוּ וּבוֹאֵנוּ,
L'-cha-yim u-l'-sha-lom,	לְחַיִּים וּלְשָׁלוֹם,
mei-atah v'-ad o-lam.	מֵעַתָּה וְעַד עוֹלָם.
Ba-ruch a-tah Adonai,	בָּרוּךְ אַתָּה יְיָ,
Sho-meir amo la-ad.	שׁוֹמֵר עַמּוֹ לָעַד:

Adonai, help us to sleep peacefully this night,
And rise with energy in the morning.
Unfurl over us a shelter of your peace,
Restore us with your wise counsel,
And take us out of harm's way.
Shield us from and remove from our midst:
Assailants, disease, violence, hunger, and anguish.
Dislodge obstacles from before and behind us,
And shelter us in the shade of your wings.
For you watch us, and pull us from danger,
You, so compassionate and kind,
Guarding our comings and goings,
Towards life and peace, now and forever.
Bountiful are you,
Protecting us, always.

Explorations

Hashkiveinu is a bedtime prayer, recited right before going to sleep.

> What is your relationship with sleep right now?
> Is there anything you that you would like to be different?

~

v'hoshieinu l'ma-an sh'mecha (and take us out of harm's way):

> Can one be strong and self-reliant . . .
>   . . . and at the same time look to be helped, even to be rescued?

> Can reaching out make us stronger, help us to grow?

v'hagein ba-adeinu (shield us):

> Is there a shield that you would like to have?
> What does it look like?
>
>> A Knight's shield?
>> A force field?
>> Wonder Woman's bracelets?
>> The canopy of a forest?

v'haseir Satan (dislodge obstacles):

The word "Satan" comes from a Hebrew verb meaning to obstruct or oppose.

Do you have any internal adversaries (or imps, or gremlins) that lead your thoughts, feelings, or actions astray?

What do these adversaries look like?
Are they their own characters, or do they speak in the personage or voices
of people known to you?

Can you approach them playfully?
Maybe tickle them, and make them laugh?
Or make their pants too big so that they keep falling down and then have to keep pulling them back up?
Or maybe tempt them with a big piece of coconut cream pie to go into another room and stop bothering you for a while?

You can also deal with them more seriously, asking them gently, but firmly, to leave.

uv'tzeil k'nafecha tastireinu (And shelter us in the shade of your wings):

> Picture some sheltering wings.
> What do they look like? Feel like?
>
> Can you pull them around you like a blanket and cuddle up?
> Or rock in them like a hammock?
>
> Or place them as the gates of a secure fort that you can hide inside?

❧

ki el shomreinu umatzileinu atah (For you watch us and pull us from danger):

What is the difference between being kept safe
And being pulled from danger?
Do they have different connotations or scenarios for you?

Is there anything you would like rescuing from:

> in this moment,
> in this time,
> in general?

Imagine being tenderly and vigilantly watched over,
Enfolded in soft, strong wings,
Holding and strengthening you
At exactly the moment you need it.

❧

> Try lifting your wings
> (your actual arms/wings, or imaginary ones)
> and wrapping them around yourself.
>
> You can also wrap your wings around someone else
> while they wrap their wings around you.

Ufros Aleinu (Shelter)

Text: Babylonian Talmud B'rachot 4b; Melody: folk

U-f'-ros aley-nu sukat sh'lo-mecha

וּפְרשׁ עָלֵינוּ סֻכַּת שְׁלוֹמֶךָ

Unfurl over us a shelter of your peace.

Explorations

Think a bit about the word *uf'ros* — to open, unfurl, fan out.

What are some things that unfurl on their own? i.e. in nature?

And what are some things that we open or unfurl in our daily lives?

~

Thinking about some of the unfurled things you just imagined,
add peace into the mix,
and try imagining different ways

peace

can be opened, unfurled.

~

Imagine for yourself a *sukkah* – a shelter – of peace.

What does it look like?
Of what materials is it made?
What color is it?
What does it smell like inside?

Does it unfurl over you, or suddenly appear?

Is it "over" you, or also around and under?

Is it fixed, or does it travel around with you?

Make a drawing – abstract or representative – of your *sukkah* of peace.

You can extend this exercise by making additional drawings and playing with different colors, materials, and shapes for your shelter. See if certain colors or shapes have different kinds of feelings, resonances for you. You might even try something unusual or unexpected, and see how that fits into the mix.

〜

Shalom, often defined as "peace", is related to shaleim, meaning "whole".

Are peace and wholeness connected for you?

〜

Try imagining yourself as a series of puzzle pieces.

Are there any pieces missing?

If they are, notice how the missing spots feel,
and whether you'd like to leave those empty spots as-is,
or whether you'd like to imagine some new pieces to fill them in.

These new pieces could be the same as the "original" pieces,
or different,
and they might change over time.

You can also experiment with interchangeable puzzle pieces
and possible empty spaces between them
and see how those different pieces and spaces feel.

〜

If you like, you can turn your self-puzzle into an ongoing art project
Of the whole and peaceful
You.

Adonai Li (No Fear)

Text: from the poem "Adon Olam", by unknown author;
Melody: Cantor Bruce Benson

Ado-nai li v'-lo i-ra   יְיָ לִי וְלֹא אִירָא

Adonai is with me, and I will not fear.

Explorations

Li is usually translated as "with me", but literally means "to me".

Do you feel a difference between "with me" and "to me"?

Can "to me" imply more of a sense of movement,
Of someone or something moving towards you, or you towards them?
A sense of approaching, of coming near?

Imagine seeing someone or something you love in the distance,
Watching it or them gradually becoming clearer, closer, more defined.

∾

Lo ira means not to fear, in the future tense.

Fear is often more about the future than the present,
more about what we anticipate happening,
than about what is currently happening.

It's not so much the spiky purple monster under the bed in and of itself,
but what we think that monster could do to us.

Take a moment to sit with your fears, and notice how they feel.
Can you see them?
Do they have a shape, a form?

29

~

Bring to mind one of your fears and imagine it as if made of plasticene or clay. (You can do this in your mind, or with actual materials.)

Hold it in your hands, and start working it.
Smoothing it, bending it, manipulating it in different ways.

See where it goes, what happens with it:

Fear, as something tactile, tangible, malleable, in your hand.

~

When someone or something is with us, we are also with them.

While receiving the gift of their presence, we're also giving the gift of our presence, our separate beings combining to produce something tangibly more than each alone.

Take a moment to feel the presence of others in your life
And your presence in others' lives
And the effervescent energy of all the presences combining.

~

Feeling a sense of God,
however we imagine God,
as being with, or to, us,
near and close,
can serve as a cushion between us and our fears.

Take a moment to picture God as a big cushy boundary between you and everything that scares the bejeebers out of you.

Allowing yourself in this moment to feel blissfully, abundantly, safe and secure.

Ozi v'Zimrat Yah
(Strength and Song)

Text: Sh'mot (Exodus) 15:2;
Melody: Rabbi Shefa Gold

O-zi v'zim-rat yah

Va-y'hi-li li-shu-ah

עָזִּי וְזִמְרָת יָהּ

וַיְהִי–לִי לִישׁוּעָה

Yah is my strength and song

And will be my sustenance and protection

Explorations

Does the word "strength" have any particular meaning for you?

> When do you feel strong?
> When do you feel not-strong?

> When you feel strong, does your strength feel large and muscular?

> Or tensile, as a fine wire?

> Or both powerful and flexible, as a great tree?

≈

Draw a picture of yourself with your strength revealed, and then, if you are able, create a pose symbolizing your strength.

≈

31

Does song give you strength?
Are there any particular songs which give you energy,
Make you feel stronger?

～

Imagine Yah as a song,

Vibrations and rhythms entering

    through your ears,
    your cells
    your core
    the fiber of your being.

～

Sometimes, when we feel a need to be stronger, we push ourselves to find the needed strength somewhere on the inside.

What if, in those times, we could instead relax and "borrow" strength from an external source?

    Imagine for a moment plugging into an energy source,
    A soft petal-y garden full of nature's verdancy
    Filling you with sweet waves of energy
    Flowing into and through you.
    Utterly calm, peaceful, and rejuvenating.

～

Think of one thing that you would like to be released from in this moment, and imagine it being lifted away in a great swoop of strength and song.

APPENDIX

Power of Imagery

Some years ago, a teacher recommended the book "Psycho-Cybernetics", by Dr. Maxwell Martz. In this book, Dr. Martz, a plastic surgeon, explains how he observed the impact of self-perception on his patients, leading him to conduct research in which he found that vividly imagining an event etches that event in our mind as memory, as if it actually happened. For instance, he found that someone afraid of speaking in public could, through their imagination, create "memories" of having given successful presentations, leading them to be a more confident speaker in the future.

The power of mental imagery is such that athletes or musicians can improve their physical performance by practicing solely in their minds. In a similar vein, Feldenkrais – a method of awareness and healing – operates through imagination as much as doing, helping our brains to begin perceiving things in different ways and informing our movements, internally as well as externally.[1]

The imagery in the explorations and exercises here are designed to do just that: allow ourselves to begin perceiving things in different ways, to see elements of our lives and beings from different angles, expand our experience of the situations we are in, and inform our motions, internal as well as external.

Texts

Jewish text (and prayer) has developed and expanded over thousands of years within a ritual framework that embraces both the ancient and the new. Almost any Jewish text can be felt as prayer. And almost any prayer can be considered as text: to be studied, contemplated, and lovingly examined, provoking thought, consideration, discussion, action, and, often, more text.

---

1 Amy Cuddy, in her research on "Power Poses", has found that the opposite is also true, that putting our bodies into positions of strength, even for short periods of time, positively alters our brain chemistry, increasing levels of testosterone (confidence) and lowering levels of cortisol (stress).

Translations

Translation is a complex art, with the translation inevitably layering the translator's interpretations and views onto the original text. With this in mind, I decided to create more interpretative, metaphorical, translations for this project, evoking the spirit of each prayer as I feel it within the context of healing. I highly recommend interacting with literal translations (available both in print and on-line) as well, and coming up with your own interpretations.

Transliteration Guide

All letters are pronounced as in English, with the following specifications:

Letter	Pronunciation
a	"ah", as in "tall"
e	"eh", as in "let"
i	"ee", as in "tree"
ei	between "eh" and "ay", like the French "é"
ey	"ay" as in "hay"
ai	"ah-ee" as in "light"
o	"oh", as in "more"
u	"oo", as in "toot"
'	"ih" as in "lit"
ch	"kh", as in "Bach"

Baruch/Blessing

Jewish prayer is largely constructed around the *b'rachah*, most often translated as "blessing". A standard *b'rachah* begins with the words *Baruch Atah Adonai*, and ends with a specific action or attribute, such as:

Baruch, blessed, are You, God, who _____ [action or attribute]

(i.e. brings bread forth from the earth; creates the fruit of the vine; makes peace.)

An alternative definition for "Baruch" was suggested by my Professor of Liturgy at the Jewish Theological Seminary, Rabbi Dr. Debra Reed Blank, who proposed translating "Baruch" as "bountiful". What I like about "bountiful" is that it evokes a spirit of plentitude and generosity as well as gratitude and praise. It also, for me, gives a sense of reciprocity with God: in blessing God, we increase God's ability to bless us (and all), which increases our ability to bless, and so forth, a continuing cycle of mutual enrichment, growth, and giving.

I believe that one of the purposes of prayer, and of our work-in-progress relationship with God, is to provide a practicum for our worldly relationships. The pathways of blessing, generosity, reciprocity, gratitude, and praise that are reinforced in prayer can continue far beyond our ritual moments, expanding our relationships with other people as well as with ourselves and all that is in the world around us.

God Language

The texts included here are Jewish prayers, which are centered around a focal point that, in English, we usually refer to as "God." According to Jewish tradition, God has a name, but one which is so powerful that it cannot be known to us. Therefore, we have in our Hebrew texts a number of what I call "use-names" for God, each with a different meaning or connotation. Translations into English can range from literal to symbolic, depending on the translator and purpose.

While using this journey, you may find it helpful to freely explore and use whichever divine names, descriptions, and imageries work best for you. To allow the prayers included here to dwell within their own resonances, the Hebrew name used for God has been kept in its original form, both in the Hebrew as well as in the English translation. In each instance, you can experiment with different names and references, using those that are most meaningful for you.

To get you started, following is a list of some traditional names for God in Hebrew, as well as some symbolic English ones.

Some Hebrew Names for God:

Transliteration	Translation	עִבְרִית
YHVH	representing the actual name of God, a word made entirely of breath consonants.	יְהֹוָה
Yah	God	יָה
Adonai	Lord	אֲדֹנָי
El, Elohim	God	אֵל, אֱלֹהִים
Elohai	My-God	אֱלֹהַי
El-Elyon	God on high	אֵל–עֶלְיוֹן
Shaddai	sustainer, provider, refuge	שַׁדַּי
Hamakom	The Place	הַמָקוֹם
Hashem	The Name	הַשֵׁם
Shechinah	The presence of God, also felt to represent the feminine attributes of God	שְׁכִינָה

Transliteration	Translation	עִבְרִית
Ehyeh-Asher-Ehyeh	I will be that which I will be	אֶהְיֶה–אֲשֶׁר–אֶהְיֶה
Hakadosh Baruch Hu	The Holy-One-Blessed-Be	הַקָּדוֹשׁ בָּרוּךְ הוּא
Ha-el Hakadosh	Holy God	הָאֵל הַקָּדוֹשׁ

Some Symbolic Names for God:

Infinite Source of Wonder

Divine One (also Holy/Blessed/Powerful/Wise/Lofty/Peaceful One)

Source of Blessing (also Source of Inspiration/Strength/Joy/Peace/Holiness/Creation/Healing/Wholeness)

Spark of Life

Creator of All

Holy Breath

Guide

Spirit of Existence

Seed of Growth

Light of the Universe

Maker of Peace

Sacred Mystery

Source of Abundance

Music

Jewish music and prayer are closely linked. Most prayers are traditionally sung or chanted: the use of musical instruments and song are described in the Torah; services in the Ancient Temple included choruses of Levites singing Psalms; and the public reading of the Torah is chanted according to an ancient system of markings known as *ta'amei mikra* (Hebrew), or *trop* (Yiddish).

The forms of Jewish music that have existed over time, and that exist today, are almost without bound, including the wide variety of traditional chants and musical styles inherent to each community, the musical influences of the many countries where Jews have dwelled over the millennia, and, particularly today, the vast array of musical styles across the world spectrum, both old and new, which have been incorporated into both religious and non-religious Jewish music performance.

For me, music functions both as its own entity, in the aesthetic, physical and emotional reverberations it can create within us; as well as a path, a tool of expression and interpretation, highlighting a moment, an event, a text or prayer, giving it additional meaning, opening our hearts, minds, and souls, helping sentiments enter into our core beings, allowing us to ascend to higher plains, to cleave with the divine. A different melody applied to a text can alter our perception of it, allowing us to see and feel it in different ways, and thus becomes a powerful tool of interpretation.

The melodies used here come from several sources, including Rabbi Shefa Gold, a remarkable inspiration, teacher and healer; Cantor Bruce Benson, who is spreading much light through his teaching and music; folk and traditional melodies; and myself. All are designed to be listened to or sung with, to be chanted, to meditate with, to float on. The musicians who recorded with me are all sparks of light, sweetness, healing, and joy.

You may find that other melodies for these texts speak to you: melodies you encounter from other sources, or melodies that come to you internally. In this, as with everything in this journey, follow your instincts, your heart, your dreams.

APPRECIATIONS

This project exists thanks to a great many people who contributed mightily of their time, wisdom, and expertise, including those of you on your own healing journeys who used this project in its beta form and helped inspire its continuation. You are my teachers, my friends, my mentors, my muses. You have not only helped bring this project into being, but enabled it to be far more than I could have ever imagined. I love and appreciate you more than words can say. Thank you.

Kelly Thiemann and Ann Bauman, who inspired this project through your immensely open and beautiful hearts, souls, and beings.

Toby Symington, Marion Werner, and Katrina Mayo-Smith of the Lloyd Symington Foundation, utter angels, who not only made this possible, but whose knowledge, wisdom, and unconditional love and support guided me at every step along the way.

Olga Louchakova, who budded the idea that this could be published, enlightened the pathway, and helped me along it.

John Schimpf and Josh Horowitz for your phenomenal ears and judgement, sweet hand-holding, utter caring, and unbelievable generosity.

Andrew Ramer, editor extraordinaire who helped bring everything together with such insight, wit, and tenderness.

Ellen Toomey, exquisite designer and envisioner who gave form and beauty to all.

Rabbi Shefa Gold and Cantor Bruce Benson, for lending the beautiful, heartfelt and deep healing energy of your music.

Avi Avital, Stu Brotman, Katja Cooper, Yair Harel, Josh Horowitz, Dominic Nuncio, Lewis Patzner, John Schott, and Cookie Segelstein, who infused and embedded your heavenly spirits and harmonies.

Carlo Bertè, for allowing me to use your breathtaking painting of Rafa'el on the cover, infusing the beginning of this journey with your transcendent vision and artistry.

Sharlene Akers, Peter Alexander, Jen Green, Leigh Korn, Chaim Mahgel, Nell Mahgel Friedman, Dorothy Richman, Keren Stronach, Eric Weiss, and Hilary Zaid, who reviewed this project at various stages and gave hugely of your extraordinary knowledge and expertise towards molding its structure and content.

Avi Assaraf, Carlo Bertè, Mendy Cahan, Yonaton Cohen, Charles Davidson, Michal Govrin, Esti Kenan, Alan Lew z"l, Marcy Lindheimer, Ruth Rainero, Debra Reed-Blank, Henry Rosenblum, J.B. Sacks, Nahma Sandrow, Beyle Schaechter-Gottesman z"l, Tina Smelser, Marty Weiner z"l, Leni Wildflower. My muses, mentors and teachers, your influence and spark is not only deep within the roots and branches of this project, but in every step of every day of my life.

The entire congregation and staff of Congregation Sha'ar Zahav, Neshamah Carlebach, Kathleen and Ernest Friedlander, Sarita Groisser, Ruth Ellen Gruber, Radley Hirsch, Mark Levine, Stephanie Rapp, Karen Schiller, Willy Schwartz, Annette Shaked, Rochelle Shoretz z"l, Simcha Weintraub, and particularly my family — Aviva & Mel, Paola & Gian-P, and my beloved Francesco & Ariel — for your inspiration, partnership, immeasurable support, advice, help and love.

This project made possible thanks to the infinite generosity, kindness, and nurturing of the Lloyd Symington Foundation.

Bio

Sharon Bernstein is a Cantor, singer, composer, Reiki practitioner, and Life Coach, with a particular interest in exploring the intersections between music, text, and prayer. A graduate of the Jewish Theological Seminary, she has been building prayer experiences for over 20 years, incorporating musical expressions from around the world, weaving new rituals, and writing music for liturgy and Yiddish poems. Since 2007, it has been her delight and honor to serve as the Cantor for Congregation Sha'ar Zahav of San Francisco.

www.ingramcontent.com/pod-product-compliance
Lightning Source LLC
Chambersburg PA
CBHW081012040426
42443CB00016B/3492